Lose Weight, Stop Overeating

Take Control of Your Appetite, Take Control of Your Life!

I0407168

David Fowler

Introduction

Over the past twenty or thirty years, a new epidemic has spread through the US, Canada, Britain and, to a lesser but still alarming extent, Western Europe too. It's not a disease in the normal sense of the word, in that it isn't caused by any viral or bacterial infection – instead, it is entirely of our own making. The epidemic in question is that of overweight and obesity.

This rise in overweight and obesity is a phenomenon which has come into being quickly and yet stealthily; it has happened during the course of most of our lifetimes, not over the past century or more. For thousands of years, human body weight had, in general, remained remarkably constant relative to height – in the US, for example, the great majority of people would gain a few pounds between their twenties and forties, then their weight would reduce again as they aged. Overweight people – and seriously overweight people especially – stood out from the rest. Look around you today and you will see that this is no longer the case.

Lose Weight, Stop Overeating

To see this another way, consider this: for all those thousands of years, most human beings consumed what they needed in order to live and function. No more, no less. Our own bodies efficiently regulated our weight and our appetites, maintaining that equilibrium between requirement and consumption. This, it seems, is no longer true.

The rise in numbers of overweight people in the US was first shown up in government data collected on a regular basis; from 1960 through 1980, there was little change in the prevalence of obesity among adults. Between the survey in 1976-1980 and the survey in 1988-1994, however, the prevalence of obesity increased by approximately eight percentage points. To put this figure into perspective, it equates to around twenty million people – a truly astonishing increase.

Since that time, levels of obesity in the US population have continued to rise. There are recent indications that the rate of increase is slowing, but the trend is still very much upwards. And, as the US leads, many other countries follow. Obesity rates in Britain, for example, are on a seemingly unstoppable rise.

Lose Weight, Stop Overeating

There are arguments about overweight and obesity, both within the scientific community and elsewhere – just how much are rates rising, are they coming to a plateau, and are the health effects of these conditions really as bad as many people suppose? In my view, such discussions may be of great interest in academic circles (and, to a great extent, to the government) – however, they mean little or nothing to an individual who wishes to lose weight, but finds it almost impossible to do.

So what has caused the increase in levels of obesity and overweight? There are various possible causes, but at root the issue is simply one of balance. If you take in more energy than your body needs to perform its regular functions, the upshot is that you will gain weight. If, by contrast, you use more energy than you take in, you will lose weight. Over the years our lives have become more sedentary, and this has doubtless contributed to the high levels of obesity which we now see. However, a rational analysis would suggest that, as we require less energy, our bodies should regulate our appetites, causing us to want and consume less. This may happen for some people, but for many it clearly does not.

Lose Weight, Stop Overeating

My aim in writing this book is to help you to lose weight by taking control of your appetite. I've divided the book into three sections; in the first, I examine what's happened to us and to what we eat over the past few decades – I believe that an understanding of this is of great importance. The second section concerns *what* you need to do to take control of your appetite and lose weight; the third is all about *how* you can do it.

What Happens – and Why

I'm hardly giving away any secrets when I say that people get fat because they eat more than people who stay slim. Yes, there are exceptions in individual cases, but for the most part this holds true. It's also blindingly obvious. And there's little doubt, in my own mind at least, that the rise in levels of overweight and obesity is caused mainly by one thing – overeating. But why do so many of us fall victim to overeating? Can't we just say no? If only it were so simple! The truth is that many of us have lost control of our appetites.

You know how it feels – we all do. That nagging feeling whenever a certain type of food's anywhere near. Just what type of food has this effect varies from one person to another; for some it's a burger, all the better with extra cheese and bacon; for others it's a big, sticky dessert; for some it may be something as simple as a particular type of candy. For me it can be meat pies, or certain candies, especially chocolate.

Whatever it may be, the feeling is the same. Whatever the food may be, you want to eat it. You may not be hungry – in fact, you're probably not – but that doesn't stop you wanting to eat. You may know that if you do eat, you'll feel bad about doing so; in fact, you may already feel bad just for *wanting* to eat. But the chances are that won't stop you. You'll eat, you'll feel bad. Next time this happens you'll most likely do the same thing. And the time after that, too.

This is a familiar feeling for an awful lot of people. But why does it happen? What makes us want to eat when we clearly don't need to? How come, when we're eating, we don't know when we're full? And why is it so difficult to just turn around and say no to food?

Eating Becomes a Habit

Many of us, as I've mentioned above, eat when we don't need to. We're not hungry, but we go ahead and have something to eat anyway. What's happened here is that we're actually eating not out of necessity but out of habit.

If you're used to having a snack between meals, you'll always tend to do this – because it's a habit you've gotten into. As with any other habit, it's not something you think about, it's just something you do. And the more you do it, the more ingrained the habit becomes. So ingrained, in fact, that it could almost be described as an addiction. And habits and addictions are both very hard to kick. So, we keep on doing the same thing, and we keep on gaining weight.

'Palatability' – a Vital Factor

I don't want to get too scientific here, but it is important to understand the idea of palatability, as that term is used within the food industry and by food scientists.

I'm sure you're familiar with the term palatable in everyday use; we use it to mean that a food tastes good, that we like that food. But this is not the same way that it's used in the scientific world. Here, describing food as palatable refers to its ability to stimulate our appetite and make us want more of it. And this is what I'll be using the term to mean throughout this book.

Within the food industry, increasing the palatability of food is a major goal; after all, the more palatable a food is, the more it will stimulate appetite, the more we'll want of it – and the more we'll buy of it. Over the years, the food industry has developed a massive level of expertise when it comes to producing highly palatable foods.

An Unholy Trinity

Palatability is all about how food engages our senses; not just taste, but pretty much the full range. How a food looks, smells, feels and sometimes even how it sounds (think of a steak sizzling on a griddle) all help to stimulate the appetite. The more this happens, the more palatable you can say that food is.

In general, the most palatable foods contain some combination of three core ingredients – these are sugar, fat and salt. For one single example, take a burger topped with cheese and bacon. The burger itself will contain fat and salt; the bacon too, along with sugar used in the curing process; the cheese is also high in both fat and salt. And it doesn't stop there. The bun (particularly if you're eating this burger in any one of our many fast-food chains) will be relatively sweet, as corn syrup will probably have been used in its production. It will probably come with a relish which also combines sugar, fat and salt.

Put all of these together and it's pretty clear that we're dealing with a very palatable piece of food indeed – add in the other senses, such as the smell of the burger, and the sensation of lifting it to your mouth, and its palatability is further enhanced. No wonder so many of them get sold every day!

From the Lab – Part One

A physician and professor in New Jersey bred two strains of lab rats. The first was bred to overfeed when a high-calorie diet was available; the second was bred to resist overfeeding. He therefore had obesity-prone and obesity-resistant rats. Although the resistant rats would overeat for a short while, they would quickly cut back their consumption, keeping their weight stable.

However, when both sets of rats were offered a creamy, rich liquid, high in both fat and sugar, they all gorged themselves on it. And, in this instance, the obesity-resistant animals did not reduce their consumption after a short time – they just went right on feeding whenever the liquid was available. Increasing either sugar or fat on their own brought about little or no change in their eating; but a combination of sugar and fat made a massive difference.

Loading and Layering

As I've already mentioned, sugar, fat and salt combine to produce highly palatable food. To increase this effect, many food producers either load these constituents onto a basic core ingredient (meat, potato or bread being examples) or layer them on top of it. Sometimes, of course, they do both.

Deep-fried tortilla chips are a good example of loading; the chip is loaded with extra fat by the frying process, in which fat replaces almost all the water. If plain tortilla chips are smothered in cheese, sour cream and sauce, that's a good example of layering. Smother the deep-fried chips and the food is both loaded and layered.

These two techniques are used extensively in many restaurant chains, and by producers of ready meals and other processed foods. They make the food more and more palatable, so we want and eat ever more of it.

Availability Soars

Another factor in our tendency to overeat is the simple availability of food. Fifty years ago, for instance, there were far fewer fast-food outlets around; if you wanted to eat, you had to either prepare something yourself, or go to a restaurant or diner and have a sit-down meal. This meant that getting something to eat was a conscious decision, which required a certain degree of action.

Today, it's incredibly easy to drop by somewhere and get food delivered to us in no time at all. There are fast-food outlets everywhere, and many of them have a drive-thru area, so you can get your fast-food fix without even leaving your car. Which means that it's easier than it ever has been to eat – and therefore to overeat. The more available something is, the more likely we'll be to take advantage of that availability.

Portion Sizes Soar Too

Yet another factor is portion size – go into many restaurants today, and the dishes served as starters are as big as main courses would have been fifty or so years back, and indeed more recently than that. And this is before you've hit the main course, which will be bigger still. Having a dessert? Check the size of that too – it'll be large. Very large.

As it is with availability, so it is with size of portions. Quite simply, the more that is put in front of you, the more you'll be inclined to eat. And the more you eat, the more you want to eat – it's a self-reinforcing cycle of behavior. And, of course, the more you eat, the more likely you are to gain weight.

Have you had enough?

When you eat, your body tells you when it's had enough, and that you should now stop eating. Or at least that's how it's supposed to work. The problem is that this happens less and less; many people seem to have lost their capacity for being satisfied when they eat. As a result, they eat too much at a sitting, and they do it again and again. You don't need me to tell you that this will lead to weight gain.

This is down to various factors; the palatability of the food put in front of us is one, availability and portion size are two more (we've just gotten used to having huge plates of food put on the table). Another factor is that much fast food and ready meals is incredibly easy to eat. As a result, we hardly notice we're eating it, so we lose the ability to tell when we've eaten enough.

The Body's Defense Mechanism Is Overwhelmed

All animals, including we humans, have an internal mechanism known as homeostasis. This is defined as the tendency for the internal environment of the body to remain constant in spite of varying external conditions, or a tendency towards health or stable physical conditions.

And it's this mechanism which served to keep our weight more or less constant for so long. Without any conscious thought or considerations, our bodies have been capable of regulating themselves such that weight is kept within certain limits; we eat what we need in order to sustain our level of activity.

But it appears that homeostasis is reeling under the assault of ever more palatable, ever more available food, served up in ever more generous helpings. It seems, in fact, as if the sheer abundance of food on offer to us has overwhelmed the body's natural defenses. And so, rather than eating as much as we need and being satisfied with that, we keep on eating more and more.

From the Lab – Part Two

This time it's not rats but humans. In a study, researchers confined adult males to a ward where their food intake could be monitored. Initially, the men were fed a diet which maintained them at their existing weight; in this diet, approximately 50% of the calories were from carbohydrates, 30% from fat and 20% from protein.

After a few days, the men were allowed to eat whatever they liked from two free vending machines. These contained a variety of entrées and snacks, giving the participants continual free access to nuts, popcorn, fries, meats, cheese, bread, tortillas, fruit, vegetables, pastries and desserts, cereal and beverages. However, they were asked to stay as close as they could to their typical eating patterns.

The results? On average, each participant ate 50% more than he needed to maintain his existing weight. It was also noted that the subjects ate considerably more fat and less protein during this period, with the typical diet containing 40% fat and 12% protein.

So, a scientifically conducted study confirms what we probably would have guessed; given the opportunity to eat unlimited quantities of high-fat, high-salt and high-sugar food, many people will do so to excess.

The Food Industry

Not surprisingly, the aim of the food industry is to sell us food. Nothing wrong with that, of course – they're in business to turn a profit, and producing and selling food is how they do that. The problem, for us at least, is that they just do it too well! Vast sums of money are spent each in year in the quest to produce food that you and I will find simply irresistible.

The techniques used by the industry have become more and more sophisticated over the years. I've already given brief descriptions of loading and layering, and how these and other things make the food we're sold ever more palatable (hyper-palatable and ultra-palatable are terms frequently used within the food industry). But it doesn't end with loading and layering; other techniques in common use include:

Making food easier to eat; much food sold in restaurants or pre-made in stores is designed to be ultra-easy to eat. If very little effort is involved in eating a plate of food, you're far less likely to be fully aware of just how much you've eaten. Foods like fried chicken wings are often prepared by injecting marinade into the raw meat; this serves the dual purpose of keeping the cooked meat moist and tenderizing it too. Both of these make it easier to wolf down without too much chewing. And, when you think about it, when you eat food like this you just don't know when you're full.

Encouraging indulgence; as Americans (and everyone else in the Western world) spend relatively little of their disposable income on food, it's easier to move away from the basic stuff and upgrade to premium products. Just as we'll pay more for sirloin steak than for rump, and more again for fillet, so we'll choose the fancier items on a restaurant's menu. These are likely to be more palatable, more indulgent – and also more profitable for the businesses that sell them.

Food as entertainment; this sits alongside indulgence. We often crave more than just food when we eat out; we want some respite from the stresses of our everyday lives, to enjoy an experience that goes beyond mere eating. And many restaurants cater for this – as an example, themed restaurants are becoming more and more popular. So we go to these places, we feel comforted, and we pay little attention to just what we're actually eating, how much we're eating or what's gone into it.

These factors all combine to create an additional effect that I've mentioned already – the loss of our ability to know when we've had enough to eat. How often have you seen people push their unfinished plate of food to one side, only to go back to it again a few minutes later? This loss of capacity to be satisfied is a key factor in the loss of control of our appetites.

Do You Know What You're Eating?

Of course you do – it's a cheeseburger with fries and a nice, healthy salad! The point is, do you know what's actually in it? Assuming you're eating it in a fast-food restaurant, you can always ask. But the staff may not be too happy about telling you. And chances are you won't ask anyway – it's just a burger, right?

Then, when you're buying ready meals in the supermarket, do you check the labels to see what's gone into them? If you do check, do you really understand what all those ingredients are? As an example, there are many different kinds of salts, many different kinds of sugar, many different kinds of fat. If the manufacturer lists these separately (as they're quite entitled to do) it's much harder to tell how much of what there is in that meal. And how many people actually check the label anyway?

Bit by bit, bite by bite, we've lost the connection that we used to have with the food that we eat. It's a connection that we need to re-establish.

Settling Higher and Higher

A good example of homeostasis in action is 'set point theory'. This says that we will adjust our energy intake and outtake to maintain a relatively constant weight. This theory also helps explain the frequent failure of diets; if

Lose Weight, Stop Overeating

you lose weight, your body is conditioned to put it back on again. It does this by slowing down your metabolism until your previous weight is re-established.

However, none of this explains how it is that so many people's weight seems to just go up and up. Clearly, this is more than a failure of homeostasis. Current thinking is that for each of us a settling point is reached, and that this is determined by a number of balancing factors. On one side are the urge to eat, and the capacity to be satisfied (or lack of it); on the other, the individual's natural ability to burn calories, plus the individual's level of physical activity. When these factors are in equilibrium, you are at your settling point.

Dieting may push the settling point down, but it is a struggle to keep it there. In addition, our constant exposure to highly palatable, highly available food is always likely to push our settling point upwards, as our urge to eat is heightened and our capacity to be satisfied is reduced.

Tried Dieting? It Sucks.

There are several reasons why dieting rarely works in the long term. The first is that dieting is almost always seen as a short-term thing – how many times have heard people say that they're going on a diet? Compare that to the number of times you've heard people say they're going to change their diet, or change their whole relationship with food. Heard those ones often, or ever? I doubt it.

Generally, going on a diet means changing what you eat for a set period; either until you lose a certain amount of weight, or for a specific length of time. Or, of course, until you get sick of it – which is what most often happens. The outcome is almost always the same though: you make no real long-term progress. You may go on a diet, lose a few pounds, feel pleased with yourself, then ditch the diet and gradually go back to eating as you did, in which case those pounds will creep back on bit by bit. Or, you start the diet, don't get the results you wanted as quick as you wanted, and give up the diet. Either way you stay the same.

A further problem with dieting is that it's invariably seen as a chore, or even a punishment. If doing something feels like a hardship, but you think that you must do it, your results will never be as good as if you're doing it because you really want to. It's all about motivation, and enjoyment too. Diets that you'll see in magazines, or online, rarely if ever stress this; they promise you results in exchange for a period of suffering. And nobody likes suffering!

Our Relationship With Food Needs To Change

I hope that, having read all I've written so far, this is the conclusion that you're already coming to. If you put all this information together, it's just about the only conclusion that you can reach. To end the chapter, here is a summary of some key points:

❖ We eat too much
❖ We eat when we're not hungry
❖ We find it hard (almost impossible) to resist certain foods
❖ We eat out of habit, not necessity

Lose Weight, Stop Overeating

- ❖ We don't know just what we're eating – and we may not even care
- ❖ We don't know when we've eaten enough
- ❖ We often feel bad about all this

Put all of that together – does that look like a healthy relationship with food? Not to me it doesn't, and that's what really needs to change.

What You Need To Do

In the last chapter, I've given you plenty of detail about why and how we've lost control of our own appetites. Now here's where we start to do something about it! In this chapter I'll be focusing on what you need to do; in the next, I'll tell you how to set about doing it.

In order to reclaim our appetites and our lives, and to change our dysfunctional relationship with food into a healthy one, we need to do several things: we need to break existing, bad habits; we need to establish new, good habits; and, first and foremost, we need to acknowledge to ourselves – and everybody else too – that the problem is ours and ours alone.

Take Responsibility

Given all that I've written about combinations of ingredients, plus of course the food industry, you could be forgiven for thinking that I've simply been arming you with a list of excuses. After all, with all these forces lined up against you, what chance can you possibly have?

Lose Weight, Stop Overeating

Thankfully, that's not it at all. Yes, I've written at some length about those forces – but this is only so you know what you're up against. Anyone can know that they find it hard to resist food, but knowing *why* you find it so hard is very important. You can't fight something if you don't what it is you're fighting; the first chapter of this book should have given you a very good idea of just what your opponent is.

So, here you are, with all those forces lined up against you. What can you do? Simple – ignore every one of them and start taking responsibility for your own actions. Nobody ever achieved anything by getting someone else to do it for them, and the situation here is no different. This book is all about taking control of your appetite and your relationship with food; if you abdicate all responsibility in the first place, then how can you hope to do that?

By taking responsibility, what I mean is that you have to recognize that you and you alone are responsible for what you eat. It's not the food industry's fault that you eat too much, for example. Sure, they do their utmost to encourage you, and you need to be aware of that – but, at the end of the day, the only person popping that food into your mouth is you. No-one else, just you.

Unless you're willing to recognize this, you'll get nowhere. You may embark on an endless succession of diets and similar programs (in fact, you may have already done just that) but it'll do you no good. One of the problems with diets (in addition to those I've already mentioned) is that they also tend to take responsibility away from you. You're doing what the diet tells you to do and, if the diet fails (as it pretty much inevitably will do) it's the diet's fault, not yours. If diets ever work, it's only in the short term. To change things in the long term, we need to change our behavior – and this starts with taking responsibility for that behavior.

The good news here is that taking responsibility does one massive thing for you. It gives you power. Real power. If you're living with a mindset that says that what you do is someone else's fault and not your own, how can you change what you do? You can't, because it's not in your hands to change it. If, on the other hand, you accept that the responsibility is yours and yours alone, you can do whatever you like. If you want to change things you can, if you're happy with things as they are then you can keep them that way – it's your choice.

When I was a kid, I always used to say "I can't help it!" whenever my mom or dad told me not to do something – it's something that all kids say. Well, my mom always had an answer for that – she'd simply say "You *can* help it!" Now, if you're still trying to tell yourself that something's not your fault, isn't that just the same? And, if my mom didn't accept that from me when I was ten years old, should you really be accepting that from yourself, now?

Get rid of old habits

'Old habits die hard' is a common saying, and with good reason. We form habits easily and kick them with great difficulty. In this chapter, I'm not concerned with how to get rid of habits, as I'll be doing that in the next chapter. Right now I'm just going to list of seven habits you need to break, and why. That's assuming you have these habits, of course – so read through the list and see how many ring true. Be honest with yourself; you've nothing to gain from not doing that.

Fast Food

This covers a whole multitude of foods, but I'm using the term here to mean the kind of stuff you grab to eat when you're a bit rushed and you want something quickly. It could be a burger, fried chicken, hot dog, pizza slice... Most likely it'll come with fries and a bucket of fizzy drink too. And maybe a dessert. Fast food outlets are everywhere – you'll find them in shopping malls, on high streets, at airports and railroad stations – anywhere you may go, it seems. Fast food is easy to buy and hard to resist – some combination!

Most fast food is high in fat, sugar and salt; as we've seen before, this is a combination which tempts us to eat more than we need, and to want even more. Burgers contain salt and fat, the buns are sweet (they're often made with corn syrup, which is high in sugar); if you have cheese and bacon too, that adds more salt and fat, and sugar too if it's sweet cured bacon – and it probably will be. Also, in many fast food places the options that appear more healthy are not likely to be so at all – just check out the levels of fat, sugar and salt in the salad dressing. Incidentally, an interesting thing to try at a fast food restaurant is to ask exactly what goes into the food you're ordering – try doing this some time and see if you get an informative reply!

Another aspect of eating fast food regularly is the lack of awareness of what you're eating. You feel a bit hungry, so maybe you grab a chili dog or some fried chicken. You don't stop and think about what's gone into this food, or about whether you really need all that intake – you just do it. Of course you do – it's a habit.

I'm not saying here that there's anything inherently bad about eating fast food – there isn't. The problem for many of us arises because doing so becomes an unthinking habit. The result is that we eat more than we need to; and, as it's become a habit to do this, we do so again and again.

Sweet stuff and candy

Like fast food, there's an awful lot of sweet stuff out there – in fact, you'll find plenty of it in places which serve fast food. But it's not desserts I'm talking about here. It's the pastries, the cookies, the cinnamon rolls, the donuts, all those things you eat in between meals. The list isn't endless, but it's long. And it doesn't seem like you're eating too much, either – after all, eating a donut or maybe two isn't like having a whole meal, is it? Maybe not, but try counting up how many you've eaten over the past week, or the past month – then think about how much it looks like!

Then there's candy too – you may have a pack on your desk, in the car, next to you at home... And, if you buy a pack of candy, can you really eat just a half or a third of it, then put it aside and not touch it again till the next day, or at least a lot later the same day? I know I have trouble doing that! The same applies to cookies; you eat one or two, then you feel like another one or two, then maybe just one more... Then half the pack's gone, and you think maybe you'll just have one last one... But then the pack's starting to look pretty empty, so you finish it off. The whole process may have taken you an hour or so.

Like fast food, eating sweets and candy like this is similar to an addiction, and it can be very hard to kick the habit. But it can be done, as long as the will to do so is there.

Eating out

When I was a kid, eating out was a real treat. We only did so very rarely, which meant that it seemed like a big occasion, something special. I don't know just how often we ate out, but from recollection I'd say no more than once every couple of months. How things have changed! In the US, the average family now eats out on a regular and frequent basis. Many of those times will be at fast food establishments, but often it'll be Chinese, Mexican or something similar.

Fast foods we've already covered, but how about the others? Surely you can't put a Chinese meal in the same category as a burger and fries? The answer, certainly in the US, is that you almost certainly can. Over the years, standard Chinese dishes have been Americanized; that in itself means that they're likely to be sweeter and saltier than they would be if you ate the same dish in Beijing. In addition, many Chinese restaurants are part of national chains; the food they serve is pre-prepared using salt, sugar and flavorings, then frozen and eventually fried in plenty of oil to serve at the restaurant. A far cry from a healthy meal that's prepared and cooked at the restaurant using fresh ingredients!

Once again, the key point here is knowing what you're eating. As with fast food, you may well find that your waiter or waitress at a Chinese, Mexican or other chain restaurant won't be able to tell you just what's gone into the food they've just brought you. And if they can't tell you, who will?

Takeaway meals

These fall somewhere between eating out and eating fast food; often, a takeaway meal will be from a fast food establishment like a burger or fried chicken restaurant. Other times it may be a Mexican or other kind of meal. As with eating these foods at the places you buy them, you're effectively passing control of what you're eating to someone else, whether it's a vast corporation or a local chef.

As with eating out, having takeaways was a rare event when I was young; it's far less so now. And, just as is the case with fast food, having a takeaway meal isn't necessarily bad or damaging in itself – it's when it becomes a habit, and something that you do on a regular basis, that it also becomes a problem.

Ready meals and processed foods

Or the non-takeaway takeaway. Many of us buy and eat ready-produced meals; it's easy to do, we have busy lives and work long hours so cooking for ourselves seems like a chore. So what's gone into the meal you're putting in the microwave tonight? Have you looked at the label? Even if you have, does it really tell you everything you should know?

Here's a neat way that food companies can get around federal laws on labeling. Let's say that something has sugar as its single largest ingredient – this may well apply to a pre-prepared dessert you've bought. According to federal regulations, sugar should sit at the top of the list of ingredients, so you know you'll be eating a lot of sugar when you eat this dessert. But if this sugar comes in more than one form – sucrose, fructose and glucose, say – then each of these can be listed separately, making the product appear to contain less sugar than it actually does.

Whether you're a hawk-eyed label reader or not, however, the fact remains that if you eat a lot of ready meals and prepared food you're handing control of what you eat to somebody else. Just like having a takeaway, then.

Processed foods sit alongside ready meals as a habit worth losing. The more processing a food has had, the farther removed it is from its original form, and the more additives and flavorings it's likely to contain. This may not seem important, but when I eat chicken, for instance, I want it to be recognizably chicken – not reclaimed, mechanically rendered stuff that's been put back together, added to and flavored to look and taste a little like chicken. And I like to know what's gone into what I'm eating, too.

Snacking

How much do you eat at your main meals in the average day? You may have a very good idea, you may have very little idea. Either way, here's another question – how much do you eat in between meals in the average day? My guess is that, even if you know pretty well exactly what you eat for breakfast, lunch and dinner, you hardly keep tabs at all on what you eat in between times.

And that's just what snacking is; little items of food that we eat because we feel like it, throughout the day and maybe the evening too. There are snacks and snacks of course; I guess you could call a piece of fruit in mid-afternoon a snack! Then there are potato chips, nachos, corn chips, candy and other sweet things... I'm sure you get the drift.

The thing here is that it's yet another example of two things – first, eating when you really don't need to and, second, eating in an uncontrolled way. Habit once again – the snack's there, the hand reaches out for it, then the process is repeated till there's no more snack. Hmm, nearly lunchtime!

Not really knowing just what you're eating – or how much

All of the habits I've mentioned above have one thing in common, and that's that they keep you from really knowing just what and how much you're eating. So for the final, overriding habit in the list, I've chosen that very lack of awareness. Because it does indeed become a habit in itself.

Lose Weight, Stop Overeating

The more that anybody lives on food that's pre-prepared, the less knowledge they'll have of their actual food intake, and the less concern they'll have about either the intake itself or their awareness of it. Lose control of your eating and appetite and you'll pretty soon lose any real interest in them too. It's a classic vicious circle.

I've seen customers at burger joints ordering a king-size burger with a large portion of fries – and a diet Coke! What kind of awareness is that of what they're eating? Do they really think that the diet drink will somehow make up for the vast pile of calories they're about to consume? I guess in such instances the diet drink order is as much a habit as the burger and fries.

How do you rate?

If you've read the last few pages and given yourself an honest assessment, my guess is that you'll recognize several or maybe even all of those habits in yourself.

Whether it's one, two, or more though, they're all habits that you need to get yourself out of. Later on I'll be going into just what you need to do to achieve that; in the meantime, here are some positive habits you could do with cultivating.

Get yourself some new habits!

Working out a list of habits you need to break is all well and good – and very necessary too – but it does have the drawback of being rather a negative thing to do. After all, you're spending your time focusing on things which aren't good, and that's never going to seem like a lot of fun!

So, to even it up a bit, here are some good habits which you should work on developing; if you take these in conjunction with shedding the bad habits you'll find it easier to do that, as these ones are in many respects a mirror image of the bad ones.

Prepare your own food

This, without a doubt, is fundamental. But then I guess you'd expect it to be – after all, I've spent a good few pages telling you to get out of habits like fast food, eating out and eating ready meals!

Lose Weight, Stop Overeating

More and more of are eating pre-prepared food of one sort or another – and we're doing it more and more often. This is caused in part by our increasingly busy lives; if you don't get home from work till late, you're far less likely to want to cook something. It's so much easier to grab a ready meal from the fridge and heat that up instead.

But preparing your own food doesn't have to be difficult or time-consuming. There are plenty of meals which will take no more than half an hour to prepare and cook, and there are plenty of books you can buy which have recipes like that in them. A simple meal like a piece of grilled or pan-fried meat or fish, served with some bread and salad, will take you maybe ten minutes to prepare – no longer than a ready meal.

I often cook a quick pasta and tuna dish – a tin of tuna steak, a tin of tomatoes, the juice of a lemon, garlic, olive oil and seasoning are all you need for to make enough sauce for two adults, and the pasta just needs to be boiled. What could be simpler? And, when I eat this, I can prepare as much or as little pasta as I like, depending on just how hungry I feel. That's just one example to show you how easy it can be, but this isn't a recipe book, so I'll leave it at that.

One other thing that you'll get from preparing your own food is a sense of satisfaction. You've done it yourself, after all. And, however simple it may have been to prepare, it still beats the process of pulling the top off a TV dinner and putting it into the microwave! And, as you've made the effort to prepare it, you'll enjoy it all the more – and you'll be more likely to savor it as you eat it, and not just wolf it down. You'll also feel a greater sense of connection with the food itself, which I think is very important.

Be aware of what you eat

This follows on quite neatly from the last bit. If you live on ready meals, fast food and takeaways, you have little or no connection with what you're eating. Put simply, it's just stuff. Highly palatable stuff maybe, but stuff all the same.

This lack of connection corresponds with a lack of awareness of what you're eating. Unless you're a real avid label-reader (and, let's face it, most of us aren't), you won't have any real idea of what's gone into the ready meal you're about to eat. And, if you have fast food or some kind of takeaway meal, you'll know even less. You'd have to ask the staff at the restaurant what's in it – and they probably won't tell you, even if they know themselves.

Having a proper awareness of what you're eating is a major part of regaining control of your appetite; once you start thinking about what you're eating, you'll become more aware of what you actually need to eat, rather than just eating out of habit.

Know when you're hungry – and when you're full

Many of us eat when we're not hungry, and eat too much as well. Why do we do this? Simple – because we've lost touch with fundamental things, like when we're hungry and when we're full. We eat out of habit, we eat food which is easy to wolf down. As a result, we never really know when we're hungry or when we've had enough to eat. Think back to those rats and their rich, creamy liquid, and you'll see we're not so far away from them.

Lose Weight, Stop Overeating

Knowing when you're hungry is really a question of breaking the habit of reaching for food when you don't need it. It's all about imposing your will over your body; as I'll be dealing with how you go about all these things in the next chapter, I'll say no more on this right here. You just need to know that it can be done and that you can do it.

Knowing when you're full is different, as it's more of a straightforward physical thing. Loss of our capacity to be satisfied is due in large part to eating food which is just too easy to eat. We wolf food down and, before we know it (and before our body knows it) we've taken in hundreds of calories. Eating food which requires some effort to eat – cutting it up, chewing it – gives the body sufficient time to feel fuller as you eat, and to eventually tell you that you've eaten enough.

For example, let's say you've prepared yourself a pork steak, which you're going to eat with some crusty bread and a salad. This isn't something that will disappear to your stomach without touching the sides – you have to cut up the meat, tear the bread, fork up the salad. You'll have time to savor the food itself and, just as importantly, your body will register that it's being fed and will give you that satisfied feeling when you've finished. And that's worth any number of unsatisfying ready meals or takeaways.

Eat at home – and do it at the table

This ties in with the previous desirable habits. We need to stop eating out of habit; to do this, we need to make eating an activity in itself, something that we do and enjoy. A special activity, not just an aside in our busy lives.

The first part of this is eating at home. Sure, there's no harm in eating out from time to time, but doing so should be a treat, not the norm. If you want to know what's in the food you eat you need to have prepared it yourself; the only way of doing that is to eat at home.

The second part is just as important. If you sit down in front of the TV with your dinner, you're treating this important aspect of your life as if it doesn't really matter at all. If a good friend calls round, you wouldn't invite them in and then sit gazing at the tube – you'd give them your attention. And that, I would say, is just how you should treat your meals. Sit at the table, turn off the TV if there's one in that room, and settle down and enjoy your meal. It's easy to do and, once you've gotten into the habit of doing it, you'll wonder why you used to eat in front of the TV!

Buy and eat things your grandmother would recognize as food

OK, maybe that should be your great-grandmother! I'm fifty-one, and both my grandmothers have long since passed – but it's their generation I'm thinking of here. To put it another way, consider how someone born before the year 1900 would view what we eat today.

Let's use a little imagination here. Try imagining your grandmother (or great-grandmother) in your local supermarket or food store. What would she see that she'd think she could cook and eat?

Well, there's fresh fruit and vegetables – those haven't changed, though the sheer variety of what's available has grown enormously over the years. I don't reckon either of my grandmothers would know what a green or red pepper or a sweet potato is, as they wouldn't have seen them in their food stores – but they'd still know that they're something you can eat. They might not have a clue how you'd cook them, or if you'd cook them at all, but they'd recognize them as food.

She'd also know meat and fish. Yes, it all tends to be highly packaged nowadays, and you won't see big lumps of flesh hanging from hooks in a supermarket. But my grandmother would know lamb from beef, chicken from pork – and she'd know ways of cooking all of them. She might be surprised at the abundance of meat in our stores these days, but that's a different story.

And I think she'd recognize a few other things. Bread, obviously (but she wouldn't expect it to be ready sliced in a packet). There's plenty of canned food that would have been common a hundred or so years back – meat, fish and vegetables – and there are other things like dairy products which have only really changed in the packaging. Milk's still milk, even if it's in a plastic bottle and not served from a churn! And dried foods like pulses, pasta and rice would all look pretty familiar to her.

But how about the great profusion of prepared stuff, which makes up the majority of the food our supermarkets sell nowadays? I think my grandmother would walk straight past all that; if she stopped to have a look she'd probably wonder why things she could prepare so easily were being sold as ready-made meals. She would quite certainly question the need for ready-made, individually-packaged meals for one or two people. All the tinfoil and plastic packs filling the freezer cabinets would look like anything but food to her. Nothing wrong with straightforward frozen meat, fish or vegetables of course, but then she'd recognize those.

When it comes to food shopping, I'm with grandma! With some exceptions, such as instant coffee, I always try to buy food which is neither processed nor pre-prepared. It's not hard to do; you just need to ignore much of the chilled stuff, keep well away from most of the frozen stuff and you're there.

A good rule of thumb, and one which works in many supermarkets, is that the stuff I want to buy (and which my grandmother would recognize as food) tends to be grouped around the edges of the store. Fresh fruit and vegetables, meat and fish, dairy products, bread – most if not all of these are normally placed around the edge.

Move on into the center of the store and you'll be more likely to find ready meals, processed and frozen foods – these are the things which are high in one or more of fat, sugar, salt and additives of various sorts. My advice is to steer clear and focus on the fresh stuff.

Reclaim your appetite and reclaim your life!

Right, that's it for this chapter. I've armed you with two lists; habits you need to drop and habits you need to pick up. Do these and you'll be well on the way to reclaiming control of your appetite and your eating. Which also means that you'll be well on the way to losing weight, and looking the way you want to look. As to how you can do these things, that's all in the next chapter.

How You Can Do It

Let me get one thing straight right now – the first part of this chapter contains nothing specific about food, overeating, or indeed overweight. And there's a good reason for this; the stuff I'm about to tell you is applicable to far more than just weight loss and overeating. It's all about the human brain and mind, the power they have and how to use that power to achieve results. I'll get around to the specifics later on, but don't expect any for the first part. Just thought I'd better let you know. And please don't skip this bit – you'll be glad you read it. OK, here we go...

The Power of the Human Brain

I'm not going to spend too long on this – it has some relevance, but only really to show you what power you have inside your own head. And I can guarantee that when you've read this, you'll be both amazed and impressed. You may well think "Does that really apply to me?" Well, I can assure you that it does. Stick with me through the next bit – it'll be worth it, I promise.

Lose Weight, Stop Overeating

Let's start with some very large numbers. We all know the names of large numbers – a million, a billion, a trillion – but it's very hard to imagine them. Can you imagine a million of anything? Here's a helping hand: a million seconds is about eleven and a half days; a billion seconds is roughly thirty-two years; and a trillion seconds is around thirty-two thousand years. Now think of a single second – it's gone just like that. That's the power of big numbers.

So why am I telling you this? Simple – to prepare you for a far, far larger number. Do you know what a googol is? It's the word which Google used to name their search engine, but apart from that it's a truly vast number. It's actually ten raised to the power of 100, expressed as 10^{100} – put another way, it's the number 1 followed by 100 zeros. Or, if you want it longhand:

10, 000, 000, 000, 000, 000, 000, 000, 000, 000, 000, 000, 000, 000, 000, 000, 000, 000, 000, 000, 000, 000, 000, 000, 000, 000, 000, 000, 000, 000, 000, 000, 000, 000, 000

Lose Weight, Stop Overeating

Any way you look at it, this is ridiculously big. Beyond comprehension even. But what's this actually all about? Well, it's about the power of the human brain.

We have about ten million brain cells; each of these is directly connected to around 100,000 other brain cells closest to it on the surface of the brain. Big numbers, but what are these brain cells actually capable of? Well, every second of your life they take in and store more information than all the computers in the world put together. Pretty impressive, huh? But that's not all.

Since the 1950s, psychologists have been attempting to estimate the power of the human brain; specifically, they are interested in how many connections one of our brain cells can have at any given moment with the brain cells that surround it. Multiply that by the number of brain cells and you have an estimate of the number of thoughts we can be entertaining at any time. Back in those days, they estimated that this number was the one I've just given above – yes, a googol. Look back up the page at it, it's a lot of thoughts for one brain to be having.

And that's just for starters. Since those early days, estimates have got higher and higher. Right now, the estimate for our potential number of concurrent thoughts is a positively frightening number – in mathematical terms, it's 2 x $10^{1,000,000}$. Put in everyday language, that's a 2 followed by almost *ten miles* of 0s – and that's a number I can't even begin to imagine, let alone understand. But that's what your brain – yes, that's your brain, my brain, everybody's brain – is thought to be capable of by people who spend a heck of a lot of time researching these things. So that's the powerhouse you're carrying around on your shoulders every day. Take good care of it, you only get the one!

The Human Mind and How It Works

So that's the power of the brain. We're on to the mind now, and it's not the same thing – but it's closely connected. I'm not about to launch into a major lecture on psychology or anything like that, but an understanding of how your mind works – and what it can do – is fundamental both to this chapter and to your ability to achieve your goals.

The mind is not an easy thing to define. It has no physical manifestation, for starters. It's connected with the brain, but it's not the same as the brain. In truth, the mind is as much a concept as a fact – but it's a very real concept. After all, we all have one, and that's about as real as it gets. That seems like a good starting point to me – the mind is not physical, but it's very real. Let's take it from there then – and keep in your mind just how much power you have in your brain as you read the next bit.

The Conscious and the Subconscious

The human mind has two parts – the conscious and the subconscious. The conscious mind makes judgments, considers and analyzes; it's the *awake* part of your mind, the part that you're using while you're reading this. Any decision you make, any course of action you embark on – all of this is the product of the conscious mind.

The subconscious is a very different thing. It doesn't think – why would it? That's a job for the conscious mind. The subconscious simply accepts and does – but what exactly does it do?

As I'm sure you'd expect, there's no simple answer to that. The best way I can put it is to say that the subconscious does everything that the conscious mind

51

doesn't do. It's also fair to say that up till now science has only begun to scratch the surface of what the subconscious can do. But here's a quick list of some things that we do know:

❖ Only about 5% of your brain capacity is conscious; the rest is devoted to the subconscious – and I've already told you how much power 95% of your brain represents.

❖ The great majority of the motor, chemical and electrical functions of your body are handled by the subconscious – that's everything from heartbeat to immune response.

❖ All memory is subconscious. In a subconscious state you can remember all manner of things that your conscious mind can't access, like where you left that thing you can't find right now.

❖ It's generally accepted that 'creative flashes', whether they're artistic or scientific, spring from the subconscious. So that could be Einstein's General Theory of Relativity, or any one of Picasso's masterpieces.

So, as you can see, your subconscious has an awful lot of power. A friend of mine described it as like having a three-year-old genie at your disposal; it's got amazing capabilities, but as it has the mind of a child, everything has to be explained to it so it can understand. Like I said earlier, the subconscious doesn't *think*, it just *does*.

Everything I've written so far in this chapter is there to help you understand the power of your own brain and mind, and particularly of your subconscious mind. Next up is where we start to get practical with this information.

How Habits Are Formed

From what I've already written, I'm sure you can guess what part of the mind is in control when you undertake any habitual action. It's not something you think about, it's just something you do – therefore, it's all taken care of by your subconscious mind.

All well and good, but how did the habit get there in the first place? After all, if the subconscious doesn't think, it can hardly initiate any action, or send you off on a course that leads to, let's say a compulsive snacking habit. The answer lies in the relationship between conscious and subconscious, and it's this relationship which you'll be able to use to your own benefit once you fully understand it. And that's not just for weight loss, as I've said before – you can persuade your subconscious to do a whole lot more than that.

So how does a conscious decision become a habit? The answer lies in two things – repetition and reinforcement. The more we do something, the more likely it is to become a habit, simply because of the repeated nature of the action. Repetition of an action pushes the responsibility for that action into the subconscious; after a while, you no longer need to think about doing something, your subconscious does it for you. And it will keep right on doing it until you tell it to stop – and that's a trick you need to learn.

Reinforcement is a different thing; it describes actions which strengthen your tendency to behave in a certain way. For example, association of two things is a kind of reinforcement. Many people who smoke, for instance, associate other activities with smoking (having a beer or a cup of coffee, for example); if they then light up a cigarette to go with their beer or coffee, that's a good example of reinforcement. Similarly, association of food with other things (a doughnut with a cup of coffee, perhaps) is reinforcing behavior.

However your habits have formed though, you need to change them.

Instructing the Subconscious

I've already said that your subconscious has enormous power, but that this is not a thinking, reasoning kind of power – which is why I described it as being like a three-year-old genie. Your personality, the way you are, the things you do – all of this is wrapped up inside your subconscious. And, if you know how to tell your subconscious what you want it to do, it will do it. That's what it's there for; it doesn't ask questions, it doesn't think about things. It just does them.

But it's not going to be as simple as saying what you want and expecting your subconscious to take this on board. And this is all the more so as what you'll be doing is getting the subconscious to change what it does. Once a habit becomes ingrained in the subconscious, it's very hard to shift. We've already seen how repetition and reinforcement create habits; now think of that happening over and over, every single day, and you'll get some idea of how deeply entrenched our habits can be. You won't shake these habits just by flicking a switch in your conscious mind.

Getting the subconscious to do what you want it to takes time and repetition. You also need to know how best to state your instructions. Remember that your subconscious doesn't think, so if you tell it to do something that requires conscious thought or consideration it won't. Why? Because you're asking it to do something it's not capable of, that's why.

In order to impose your conscious will onto your subconscious, you need to keep it simple, direct and positive. Repeating a phrase like "I want to be slim" over and over will have no effect whatsoever; your subconscious may understand the concept of slim, but it will have no idea of how you want to get there, or exactly what you want it to do.

What it will understand is a mental picture of how you want to be, what you want to be doing, and so on. This is the process of visualization which, if used well, can be very powerful indeed. The other thing your subconscious can get to grips with is affirmation; in other words, regular repetition of how you want to be. The subconscious works best with emotion rather than reason, so giving it positive feelings and emotions to use is a very good way to communicate with it.

Visualization and How to Use It

Visualization is very powerful – but there are certain things you need to know in order to make it work for you.

First, it won't work all by itself. By this I mean that simply visualizing something is not enough to make that thing happen – you'll need to do things as well. I've met people who think that visualization means simply thinking about something, then waiting for it to happen; they're also very cynical about the whole idea. But their skepticism is based on an incorrect view of visualization. By visualizing something that you want, you are effectively asking your subconscious to find a way of making it happen for you. Your subconscious will help you all it can, but any actions will be down to you.

Second, you need to be certain and specific about your vision, and picture it to yourself strongly. Specific because your subconscious won't know what to do with vague ideas, but it will understand a precise image. You also need to do this regularly (I'd suggest at least once a day, preferably more) to implant the image firmly in your subconscious.

Third, you do need to be realistic in what you visualize – but don't take this to mean that you should be safe or lacking in ambition. For example, I've never been a good tennis player, and I'm 51 years of age – so no matter how hard I might try to visualize myself holding aloft a trophy at Wimbledon or Flushing Meadow, it's not going to happen. On the other hand, I could picture myself playing at a level well above where I am now; along with the necessary practice, this would improve my game. In this instance, my visualization would spur me on to practice more and give me the belief that I can play better than I currently do.

Finally, and perhaps most importantly, what you visualize MUST be positive in its nature. So, for weight loss, focus on a slimmer you – don't think about the weight you want to shed or the fat you want to get rid of. Looking at the negative side of the equation will not be effective; in addition, you actually run the risk of having an opposite to that which you intend. If you wish to enjoy good health and fitness, you should picture yourself doing just that, not focus on the ailments you want to avoid.

When you visualize, it's also helpful to have words and phrases to go with the images, as this will help to reinforce them in your subconscious. If you do this, though, you need to make sure that any words you use are firmly in the present. In other words, think and talk of yourself as you want to be as if that is already the case, not as something that you desire. This way, both the image and the words will be instilled into your subconscious as facts, not mere wishes.

Some Visualization Examples

Naturally, visualization will be different for each person; only you can know just what you want, and I'm not going t try to tell you. But I can give you some more general examples of the types of images that will work well when weight loss is your primary goal.

Lose Weight, Stop Overeating

An obvious example is clothes size. Think of the size you want to be wearing (how this is measured will depend on where you are and whether you're a man or a woman). You can visualize this in more than one way – you could picture yourself buying clothes in your desired size, trying them on and feeling how well they fit; you could see yourself in your own bedroom, with a wardrobe filled with clothes of your desired size, choosing what to wear that day.

Another good thing to picture is your weight. First, you need to decide what your ideal weight would be (the chances are that you already have a pretty good idea of that). Then you could visualize yourself stepping onto weighing scales, and seeing them show your perfect weight – the person you picture will be the you that you want to be.

Or you could picture yourself on the beach, looking slim and great in your swimwear. A variation on the clothes theme, and potentially a very powerful image.

On a different note, you could imagine yourself walking calmly past a table covered in the foods that you find hardest to resist. If you do this, though, make sure that your focus is on how easily you can walk by this food, and how great it feels that you can do so, and not on the food itself.

How to Visualize

Different people use different techniques when it comes to visualization. I'll describe one which is favored by many, including myself.

First, get yourself properly relaxed; this is the best state for communicating your desires to your subconscious. You can be sitting in a comfortable chair, or lying on your back on your bed or the floor – there's no right or wrong here, do what works best for you. Breathe slowly; with each out breath, feel your body relaxing, all tension slowly draining away. If you like, you can do this bit by bit; the first few out breaths relax your feet, the next few your legs, then your hips, and so on. Your limbs should start to feel heavy and warm; you will also feel yourself sinking into your bed, chair or the floor. But you need to keep your mind active, otherwise you'll go to sleep.

Once you're fully relaxed, bring the image you desire into your mind. Picture it as fully and as strongly as you can;

enjoy the image, let it make you feel good. As the subconscious is not a thinking thing, it responds better to emotion than to reason – the more you enjoy your image, the better it makes you feel, the more impact it will have on your subconscious.

At the same time as picturing your image, repeat to yourself the phrase that you associate with it. Taking the clothes size example above, you might say something like: "I have a wardrobe full of size x clothes – they all fit me perfectly." Note that my x here represents the size you'd like to be, not any actual clothes size!

Repeat this for as long as you like, savoring and enjoying the feeling that it gives you. Then, if you have another image and phrase which you wish to use, move on to this one, repeating it in the same way as you did the first. And so on; there's no limit to the number of images you can picture, it's entirely up to you.

Once you've done all the visualization you want to, you can stay in your relaxed state as long as you wish – relaxation is very beneficial. Once you're completely done, bring yourself gently back into the here and now, becoming aware again of things around you, waking up fingers and toes, stretching gently. Once you've done that, have a good stretch, a yawn, and let you breathing return to normal. You will feel at ease with yourself and with the world; regular visualization will help you to attain the goals you have set yourself.

Visualization is, as I have said, very powerful. It is used by many very successful people in all walks of life – business, sport, the arts and so forth. Do it regularly and well and you will begin to feel its benefits.

Affirmations and How to Use Them

An affirmation is a simple statement, which you can repeat as often as you wish – it's not necessary to get yourself all relaxed for this, so it's easy to do it as many times in a day as you want to. Affirmations can be used along with visualization; they help to reinforce the images you use and to drive them deep into your subconscious.

Similar rules apply to affirmations as to visualization. Your statements should always be set in the present, not the future; they should always be phrased in a positive way; they should be kept as short and simple as possible; and they should feel right for you. In addition, you should try as much as possible to create a feeling of belief that your affirmations can be true.

Some people like to use the second person for their affirmations; in other words, rather than starting with 'I', they use their own name, as if talking to themselves. Whether you choose to do this or not is, of course, entirely up to you.

When choosing your affirmations, always think about exactly what it is you want, then tailor the statement to reflect that. Never focus on what you don't want, as this won't have the desired effect.

Here's a good affirmation example, taken from my own life. I was aware that I had a tendency not to finish things that I started; not always, but enough that I wasn't happy about it. I realized that to change this I had to change the way I see myself, and let this sink into my subconscious. So I used this affirmation:

I complete what I start, always and without exception

I would repeat this to myself, visualizing at the same time the sense of satisfaction and accomplishment I would feel on completing each task I had started. And, over time, it became natural for me to carry any task through to completion, and not leave anything part done. Note that the affirmation focuses on the positive (completion of tasks) rather than stating that I do not leave things unfinished. That's a very important point which I'll go into more a little later.

Here are some affirmations that you might find useful for weight loss – remember that these are just examples, and you should always devise and use affirmations that are exactly right for you.

I weigh less than nnn pounds.

I eat three meals each day; this is all I require.

I am slim and fit; I exercise regularly to keep this way.

I look terrific in a bikini!

I have a great figure; I am totally happy with my shape.

I walk calmly past fast-food joints.

Lose Weight, Stop Overeating

I always eat healthily, and in moderation.

I prepare my own meals – I love doing this!

Mealtimes are special times in my house.

As before, you can see that each of the affirmations is positive, focusing on how you want to be and what you want to do, not on the things you want to put behind you.

Remember that all the visualization and affirmations you use must be right for you; if they're not, you can repeat them as much as you like but they'll have no effect. And that's why I've only suggested a few possible ones as general guidelines. You are your own person and you're unique, so you need to decide what's right for you.

Always Positive, Never Negative

I really can't stress this too much. Everything you visualize, every affirmation that you use, has to be positive. It has to make you feel good, not only about what you're visualizing or affirming, but about yourself too.

Lose Weight, Stop Overeating

That's why I've said how important it is to focus in on feeling good about things in your visualization. If you visualize good, happy feelings, you're passing those thoughts and ideas right on to your subconscious, and it will pick up on the emotion you're expressing.

If you picture negatives, or use negative phrases in your affirmations, you are in effect focusing your mind, and therefore your subconscious, on the things that you don't want. If you do this, it doesn't matter how much you say you don't want them, the image or thought is of the thing you don't want. When a sports star (let's go with tennis and say Raphael Nadal) is about to play a major final, do you think he visualizes the bad feeling he'll have if he loses in order to get motivated? Of course not – he'll visualize winning the title. In his mind he'll be playing the winning shot, hearing the reaction from the crowd, lifting the trophy and drinking in the applause.

As a practical example, let's take the affirmation I gave a little earlier:

I complete what I start, always and without exception.

Lose Weight, Stop Overeating

Now, maybe I could have phrased that differently, like this:

I never leave things unfinished once I've started them.

On the face of it, there's not a whole lot of difference there – the two sentences mean much the same thing. However, you have to remember that you're dealing with your subconscious here; and it doesn't think or analyze, it will focus on what you're telling it, on the images you're giving it.

In this case, the image is one of finishing things – and, to make sure the message hits its target, I would emphasize it with thoughts of how pleased I'd feel about completing stuff. If I'd used the second example as an affirmation, it just wouldn't have worked. First, I'd be focusing on leaving things unfinished, so that's the message my subconscious would pick up on. Second, I wouldn't be able to conjure up those great feelings about seeing things through to the end – you can't generate positive feelings from a statement that's negative.

A final point here. I've already said that in many ways your subconscious is like a three-year-old genie. If you want a three-year-old child to do something, would you give him a list of things you don't want him to do, and hope that he'll then do the thing you want him to? Of course not – you tell him clearly and specifically what you want him to do. Well, that's how you need to treat your subconscious.

So, as the old song goes – accentuate the positive, eliminate the negative, latch on to the affirmative... Always.

Believe in Yourself!

The final part in the jigsaw of visualization is belief. You really need to believe that the things you're instilling into your subconscious are possible; if you have doubts about it, it'll never happen.

It may be that this is something that you'll need to work on. You may find it relatively easy to picture yourself as you'd like to be, but believing you can really be that way might be a whole lot harder. So you'll need to work at it – try telling yourself that plenty of other people have done what you want to, so why not you?

Another way around this is to do it in smaller steps. Let's say, for example, that your ultimate goal is a certain clothes size, and that to get there you'll need to come down several sizes. If doing this seems like an impossible dream, why not see yourself one or maybe two sizes slimmer? This should be a lot easier to picture and to believe.

Once you've got there, of course, you can see what now seems believable. Maybe you'll have the confidence to go further this time, maybe you'll do the whole thing one size at a time. There's no right or wrong here, except of course what's right for you.

How Long Will All This Take?

Unfortunately, that's something that I can't answer. We're all different, and it will certainly be the case that some people have habits that are more profoundly embedded, and therefore harder to shift.

I have a friend who gave up taking sugar in his coffee a few years ago. He didn't use any of the techniques I've talked about, he simply stopped putting any sugar in the cup. He reckoned it took him about three months before he felt like it was natural to make himself a cup of coffee and not put any sugar in there. So, he kicked a habit, and it took him some time to get to the point where he no longer missed that sugar. You can take two things from this; first, the habit he lost wasn't a real serious one; second, he did it without the help of visualization or affirmations. So on the one hand it was easier than what you're about to do, but on the other he didn't have the help that you will. For me, visualization is what really makes the difference.

I have used visualization and affirmations myself and felt positive, beneficial effects from them within a month or two. This doesn't mean that what I wanted happened in that period of time, simply that I had set things in motion and could feel that this was the case. I've written a little more about myself and my experiences at the end of this book. But you can be sure that if I didn't believe that this works, I wouldn't be advising anybody else to try it!

The more you want something, the more likely it is that you'll achieve it – and that you'll start seeing results quickly. But don't fool yourself, and don't expect too much too soon. If you're seriously overweight or obese, it will take you a considerable amount of time to lose the weight you want to lose. Unless, of course, you opt for a near-starvation diet or a gastric band – and would you really want to do that?

The key thing, I think, is that you should start to feel the effects of your visualization and affirmations within a couple of months of starting. Your subconscious will begin to change your behavior, and pretty soon you'll find that you can resist previously irresistible foods, and that your eating habits are changing for the better.

So start making things happen for you; over time you'll start to feel some positive effects kicking in. Once this happens, make sure you stick with it. In fact, redouble your efforts – this is one good thing you really can't have too much of.

A Final Word

I hope that this book has been helpful to you, and that it's also inspired you to make that positive change in your life. As I've said, I know that the techniques I've described work, because they've worked for me in various different areas. They've also worked for other people that I know.

I know that you can achieve whatever you set out to achieve; you just need to believe in yourself and in your ability to do what you set out to do. Visualization and affirmation are great ways of instilling that belief in yourself. Remember, they're used (and have been used for centuries) by many, many highly successful people in all walks of life.

I'll finish off with a final thought, courtesy of Henry Ford:

"Whether you think you can do a thing or not, you're right."

Take control of your appetite, take control of your life – you'll be glad you did!

A Bit About Me...

As I've written a book on weight loss, you may well be wondering to what extent I've ever experienced problems like overeating or overweight. So, as a kind of epilogue to the book, here's a bit about me.

I was born in 1960, so I'm fifty-one years old at the time of writing. I'm five foot nine inches tall and weigh around 170 pounds. This varies a little, as you'd expect. Sometimes it's a little more, sometimes a little less. I don't weigh myself that often!

I guess that doesn't sound overweight, and I guess it's not. According to the Wii Fit we have at home, I should only weigh about 150 pounds – I reckon that if I did I'd look like a garden rake! For me, 170 feels about right.

So I'm not overweight now, but my weight in the past has gone up to around 185 pounds. Again, this isn't seriously overweight for my size, but it felt like too much to me. And, when I was that weight, I recognized in myself a lot of the traits associated with overeating. I'd eat more than I required, more often than I needed to; I've never been particularly sweet-toothed or a fast food junkie, but I was eating too much in the way of pre-made foods (as I said at the start of this book, meat pies are a weakness) and chocolate too.

To get where I am and stay there, I use the techniques of visualization and affirmation I've described here – so yes, I do practice what I preach! I've found over the past year that this has helped me to first attain and then maintain my weight and physical shape the way I like them to be. I eat healthily, and not to excess; I get a reasonable amount of exercise too. I guess if I wanted to be super-fit or super-slim I'd need to do more than I do – but I don't. I'm happy with myself as I am.

Which, when it comes right down to it, is how we all want to be.

www.ingramcontent.com/pod-product-compliance
Lightning Source LLC
Chambersburg PA
CBHW060205290526
45789CB00003B/1167